A VERY SHORT NOTE ON THE AYUSH SYSTEMS

WITH A LIST OF CLASSIFIED HERBS COMBINING THE SYSTEMS

VAIBHAV SUNDER

Made with ♥ on the Notion Press Platform
www.notionpress.com

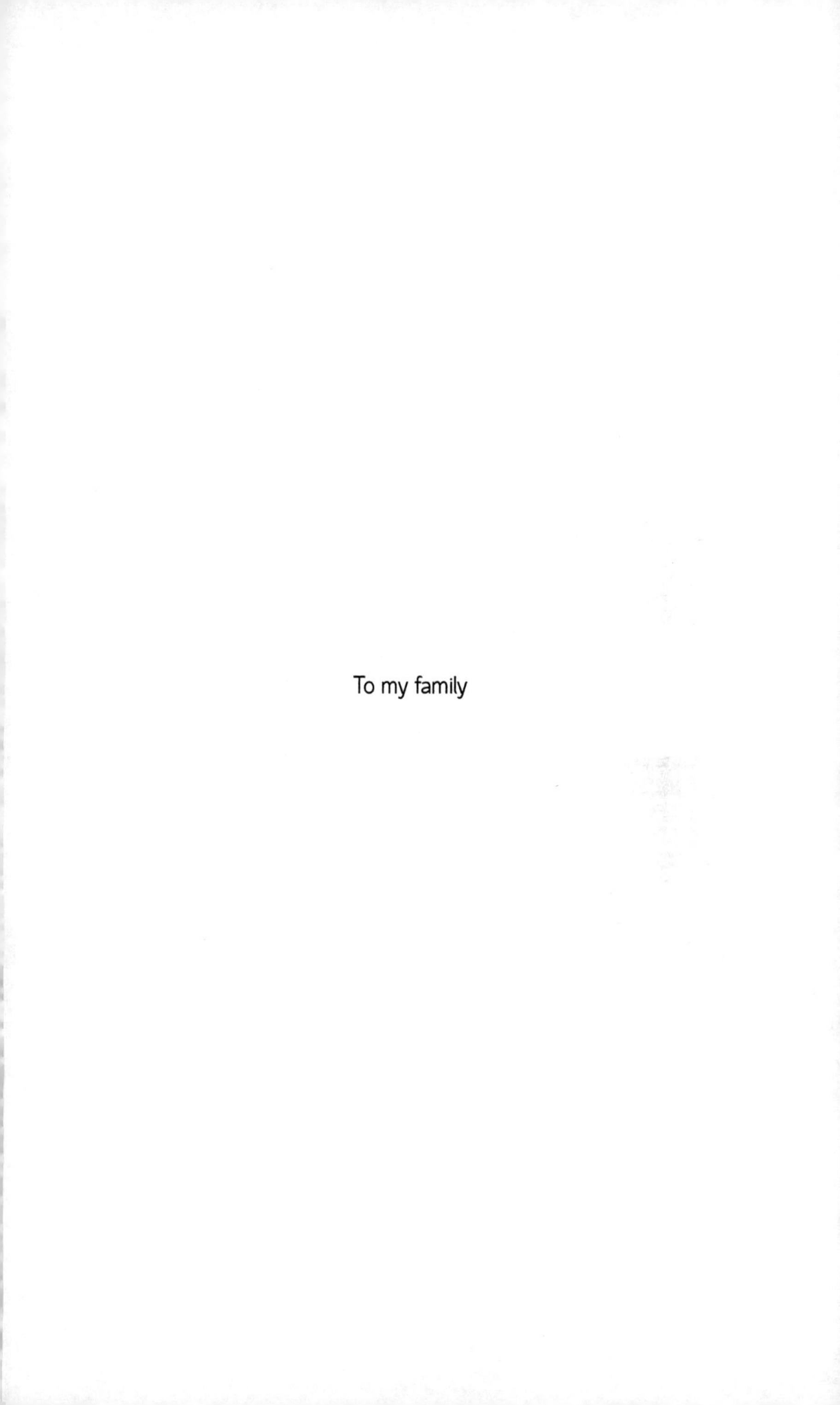

To my family

Contents

Foreword

"About astrology and palmistry: they are good because they make people vivid and full of possibilities. They are communism at its best. Everybody has a birthday and almost everybody has a palm." Kurt Vonnegut, American satirist

"I believe in astrology as much as I do in genetics." Quincy Jones

"He is a poor astrologer who pretends by the stars to point out another's destiny, and yet does not know his own." Jaafar

"Astrology reveals the will of the gods." Juvenal

Preface

The scope of this book is to felicitate the reader with the core and crux of how to apply Jyotish and Ayurveda. At first those who are knowing of basics of both Astrology and AYUSH or are familiar with it's core principles are my target audience. Even though I try to write the some references to how to start from the beginning, and then lead them towards an orientation of how to apply them or rather can apply them. More for self-realization and spiritual strength then, for only practice or professional conduct.

Preface

Acknowledgements

I am thankful to all the authors I quote that helped me shape this text

Prologue

Astrology or Jyotish, is nearly one and the same. Jyotish is one of the six critical organs to learn before trying to understand the Vedas. Jyotish is the eyes. It seeks to provide a vision to view something Universal. A good way to begin a deeper study of the Vedas and medical understanding of the world is Atharva Samhita Vidhan by Keshav Dev Shastri and Mandan Misra.

Astrology then, is a tool to understand what your Will in the sense of Theos or Div and their impact on the body is. This means although people spend decades understanding what the meaning of life is, many try to take support of Usuli (Urdu/Farsi word) or traditional methods to try to speed up that process. Today, resources are scarce for most people and time is even costlier. Without a strong disposition to be able to work with the world or by religious methods, many people in larger cities resort also to Hatha Yoga, Tapas and sometimes psychoactives to try to burn away acquired Karma or material philosophy taught in Secular educational institutions. Countries like Russia or the Mohammaden realms, always keep a Church or religious curriculum inside the educational system. In India, although there are attempts to revive the Gurukul system, the problem is that such students will not be economically aggressive in a predatory culture that is inborn due to the pace and evolutionary demands of India. I hope those who have some time, can use this book to jumpstart in their paths.

CHAPTER ONE

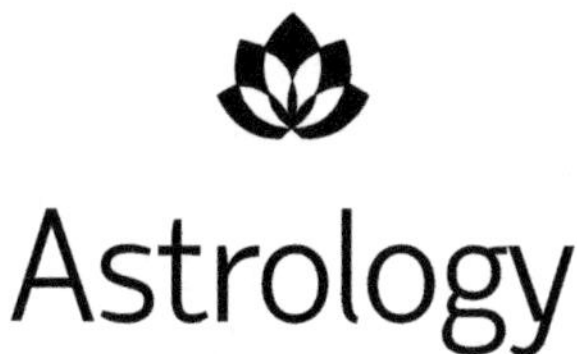

Astrology

Astrology means that there are certain dispositions of certain abstract ideas that are created by certain elements that are represented in planets and the zodiac. In ancient times, there was a culture of pith, which is universal. In Greek, the philosophers spoke a very different language, filled with complexities such as declensions and others. Today, language is easier to acquire but the amount of data that has to crunched is nearly infinite. Thus mostly, people do not seek the correct and personal path for a very long time.

Flux of existence, a book by Vaidya Upendra Digambar Dixit clearly explains the Vedic worldview of how we move internally from universal points of view. One can read of people advertising being able to give Deeksha, Shaktipat or Kundalini knowledge based on a commercial transaction. This is dangerous territory. Although the author has read of these in detail and had certain strong life changing epiphanies, later I had to incline with the same non-material, secular principles that these things must not be discussed. Because they will cause Kleshas or Dvesh to the will of those who have not decided as souls to give themselves these glimpses of direct experiences, as discussed by Adi Shankaracharya in Drig Drishya Viveka.

This book is a manual to bring personal religious revival, using the mass available tools to the simple world - by referring to books, ideas and methods that lead the person himself or herself to certain experiences that will then bring integration of the idea of the world and the self. I admit, by now I do not like the idea of groups and mass movements, and a near ascetical lifestyle is required to achieve these. But using Sadhanas and personal time available, a person in due diligence can lead to these experiences for certain. I for example, was struggling to graduate in English in Delhi University when events happened around me. Today, the world is mired in my personal life, but constant push ahead leads to material progress also and the events of spirit repeat themselves. I believe strongly, that the one thing to resolve by is, the immaterial world in itself, never loses or destroys. So if nothing is lost, the person can keep moving to the previous experience in his life, and moving ahead, the people, projections may change, but the soul will replace whatever is lost and march to whatever it is seeking. It can be hinted to by way of Akashic records. It is much like a grand macro snake and ladders, except things get emotional, damaged, lost and redeemed over time.

CHAPTER TWO

The Stars of the Ancient Eyes

The old and time-tested system of observing events and relationships begins with the indoctrination of Astrology or Jyotish, In the beginning, it is certain that our ancestors lived nomadic and tribal lives. Here the tribal is to connote the system of pre-agrarian. There are some views that will be viewed by looking at the following map.

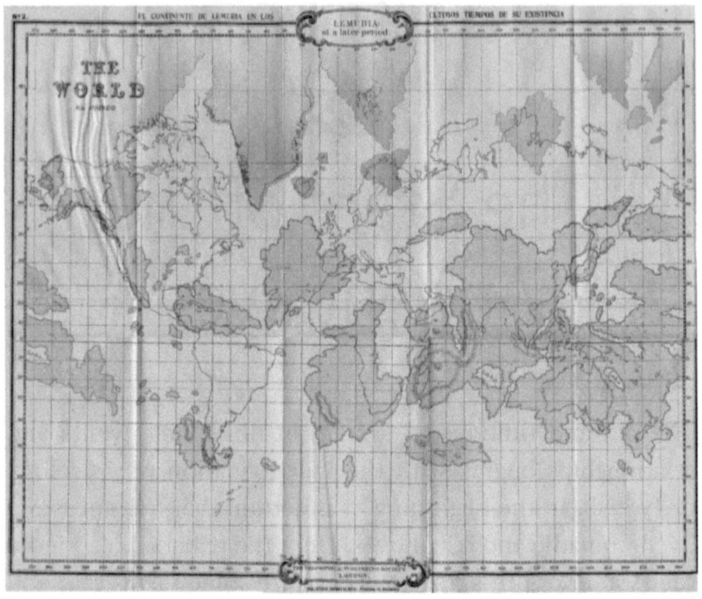

Map of Lemuria superimposed over the modern continents from William Scott-Elliot, The Story of Atlantis and Lost Lemuria.Created: 1896

More of this can be read in Theosophical literature.

CHAPTER THREE

The literature ahead

Now, in those times, not only did the evolutionary scientific vision of people looking at the night sky and creating myths happen, but the belief in the cyclical deluge and the ancestors being privy to more advanced knowledge has to be believed before delving into Jyotish.

Then, there are some key texts I will point to understand the spheres of Astrology, below -

Sagar Publication located at Janpath, New Delhi, India has a strong collection of preliminary books to read on Astrology

There is an organization called 13 Moons, you can find it on 13moons.com, here there is a basis for a futuristic almanac and ephemeris, where 13 lunar cycles can be fixed into one solar year.

To see the basis for universal Astrology between the Vedic and the 13 moons doctrines, Michio Yano from Japan has written a historical text called Esoteric Buddhist Astrology. When you read it, you will see that before Semetic cohesion was created people believed in a 9 house Astrology. This can be re-affirmed and better understood by reading Prash Trivedi, published by Sagar Publications, who also agrees that the 9-house astrology, instead of the 12-house astrology today, existed. In his book on

Nakshatras, he points to the fact that the zodiac earlier, ended at Jyeshtha Nakshatra, or the asterism within Scorpio.

Tibetan Astrology books are available on Men Tsee Khang, a Dharmshala, Himachal Pradesh, India-based organization that is associated with Tibetans and leads to correct Chinese thereafter, if you come from the West of the Tibetan views.

Then read the I Ching or any good book on Chinese Astrology, keeping Michio Yano in memory.

CHAPTER FOUR

Why build a personal Horoscope

After you have understood the philosophy and the breadth and divisions of astrology. It would be time to see how the material self that you inhabit is enforced upon the will of the divine realm.

Although I can point to P.V.R. Narasimha Rao's book Vedic Astrology, there are some details I offer over and above what he says. His book is available freely over the internet along with software, again free called Jagannath Hora. That has the most detailed workings of Vedic Jyotish for now.

Spiritual Viewpoints

Do not view your chart in only one division. For one, D1 and D9 are the two charts that are looked at by Astrologers along the present tense chart, called Mundane Charts, these show the asterisms at the present moment. To work beyond the D1 and D9 is the quintessential feature.

To understand Divisional Charts, first, know that those Nakshatras in the Zodiac circle that were rising above the head at the point of birth are reflected in D1. Now to form another basic view, the Lunar cycle is of 28 days, this has been pointed to in Greek and Hebrew literature as a

Metonic cycle where 19 years of lunar cycle creates a division. The 28 days are alluded to in the cycle of women and their movement in the womb. Nitya Devis are 16 in number and makeup one fortnight with one Devi as the complete occulting 16th. Then, the rotation of the Sun is alluded to as the second cycle, all religions including Christianity agree that the Equinox, two solstices hold very special value for the divine realm. And they make up as abstract stations when the Solar cycle is looked at. Every 11 years a sunspot cycle completes, where the Sun releases solar flares. The third cycle is the slowest and outer to the Earth is an imaginary belt of the zodiac. It can be viewed in more detail by looking at an armillary, that was created and is still sold at many antique shops and online as a network of spheres that rotate around the earth and even the Solar system, as envisaged today. Because we are less knowledgeable about the events outside of our Solar system, for now, we use this abstraction. Where Saturn, Neptune, Uranus, and Pluto were the farthest. Pluto has since been removed as a planet due to its small size. The Vedic view of a Vishnu Nabhi, where our own Solar system is also revolving around a center is the farthest reach point. Wait for Amazon's Deep Blue, Musk and others to commercialise the space to see more elaborations.

CHAPTER FIVE

Creating your own views

When D1 and D9 are surpassed as zooming into the first impression made upon the native since his birth of D1, there are about 10 standard Divisions, talked of. Each of these divisions is used for some purpose, for example, D10 is looked at for Career. But on standard software, you can view division charts - if your birth time is accurate and birth time rectification is done if not, up to D60, and the highest four divisions being D81, D108, D144 and D160.

These divisions can be analyzed for understanding how precise events cycle our world from a very microcosmic viewpoint.

Creating your own Karma with abstractions to able-ly dissolve

In the Jaimini sutra, there is talk of Chara Karakas. These are intuitively inclined if you are religious and follow a correct Sadhana. Although as per the main book of Jyotish B.P.H.S. by Parashar, all Karakas are fixed. As per Jaimini, his disciple, and his book, they can be viewed as variants also. And this variant set of planet representations of from which planet the Father, Mother, Spiritual teacher, Wife, Enemies and Kids, Brothers are to be seen changes. It also changes with each Divisional Chart.

And thus, by looking at very fine views, such as D60, and its Karakas it can be ascertained who the universal and majoritarian benefics are. Then, their Sadhanas can be carried out and inter-life Prarabhdas or life Karmas be dissolved.

CHAPTER SIX

Working with Planets

Rahu

Rahu represents the aspect of Maya or illusionary life with false impressions. It is the upper node of the two shadow nodes, the other being Ketu. Some associate Rahu with being the shadow of Saturn, and other schools with the shadow of Mars. They are both correct views.

Rahu if in the 9th is not considered very favourable by the ancestors, such as Garga Muni. However, with the passage of time, there are bigger evils to deal with by now a 9th house Rahu from the Lagna or Ascendant is called possibly acceptable. The most widely read native with such a placement is J.Krishnamurti who had Rahu in 9th in Aquarius. The analysis of the chart is in Prash Trivedi's book on Rahu and Ketu.

The impact of Rahu being favourable then, is viewed by looking at the 80-year Dasha chart called Ashottari and not Vimshottari which is a 120-year cycle Dasha and keeps Jupiter as Pradhan or the main benefactor.

The impact Ketu in 9th is the opposite. That is, it makes the native very favourable for benevolently addressing religious issues by Jupiter or Spiritual leaders.

Working with Jupiter

An exalted or high Jupiter will always allow the person to address the problems of lives even outside religions correctly. That is because the native is dipped in correct or Orthodox beliefs and will not resort to Totkas or Upayas, and sometimes due to past Karma even Sadhanas.

Working with Venus

It is a cold element and when favourably placed brings comfort. When very active along with Moon, Yogini Dashas should be worked to see the correct and depth of events,

Working with Mercury

A very strong Mercury allows working with the king of Dashas of today's times it is called the Kalachakra Dasha system. It is mostly associated with Tibetan Buddhism and mostly all forms of Buddhism due to its reflection of Intelligence and its driving maps.

CHAPTER SEVEN

The Herbs in the Current Light of Existence

In Ayurveda, the worldview is built on a four-fold division of time or Kal. It is-

- Chhand Kal
- Mantra Kal
- Brahman Kal
- Sutra Kal

In Tantra Yukti -

- Components of quest - Nyaya
- Pratigya - Hypothesis
- Hetu - Cause
- Udaharan - Example
- Upnaya - Correlation
- Nigama - Conclusion

This division is the basis for seeing the world today. With the present being associated with Sutra Kal.

Vedic rituals and Homs being a key factors in reminding us of the division. A modern text that still tries to assimilate ancient knowledge of the Fire altars into Astronomy and Astrology is a book on the Rig Vedic Altars by Subhash Kak.

Dravyaguna is the material basis for understanding Ayurvedic literature and it's use of substances. These have to be understood in the above ecosystem. So, today although we lead more comfortable lives than our ancestors, our intake of elemental externals is very complex. That is because radiation from electronics and pollutants in the water and air make not only toxic compounds to enter our systems of the body, they also inject complex compounds instead of simple mixes of elements in the old ages.

The industrialized world is unsuitable for the use of AYUSH medication is a bare fact. If one lives in an agrarian and rural land, then Unani and Ayurveda will work in India, and elsewhere. If the compounds that are in intake reach Industria admixture, use Homoeopathy. If you concur with Chinese lifestyles, then TCM and Acupressure and Acupuncture will work. If there is a desire to translate anything from or to Chinese sciences, use Tibetan views first and then reach into the lenses of Chinese.

A chart for use in Unani medicine which is the basis for Structural Semetic and Abrahamic doctrines is given below -

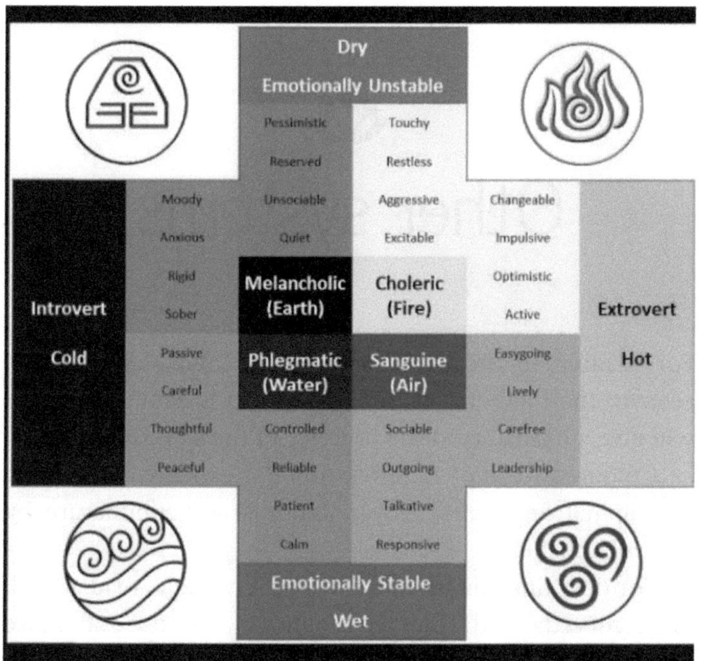
Dry
Emotionally Unstable
Pessimistic
Reserved
Unsociable
Quiet
Touchy
Restless
Aggressive
Excitable
Moody
Anxious
Rigid
Sober
Changeable
Impulsive
Optimistic
Active
Introvert
Cold
Melancholic
(Earth)
Choleric
(Fire)
Extrovert
Hot
Phlegmatic
(Water)
Sanguine
(Air)
Passive
Careful
Thoughtful
Peaceful
Easygoing
Lively
Carefree
Leadership
Controlled
Reliable
Patient
Calm
Sociable
Outgoing
Talkative
Responsive
Emotionally Stable
Wet

Unani

CHAPTER EIGHT

Other systems

For reading in detail on Acupressure and Acupuncture, refer to the following map book, which is economical and will give a headstart to the practice of the sciences.

Coloured Atlas of Acupressure: Reflexology, Shiatsu, Su Jok, Spinal Segments, Dhyan Mudras & Acupuncture by B.Jain Publishers

For detailing key unique sides of Ayurveda, read a book on Ayurveda on Tongue Diagnosis, its use of Pulse classifications, and good practice of Yoga every day such as Neti, and Basti among others. For Siddha medicine, the worldview of the body as a vehicle of the microcosmos is essential and then one can lift to the concepts of Astral bodies and Antahkran.

To end the phase of AYUSH subjects I point to a book called Planetary Herbology by Michael Tierra that will save a lot of time in trying to integrate all these subjects in Astrology and AYUSH into one.

It outlines the basic nature of all herbs and systems such as European herbs, TCM, and Ayurveda, and divides them according to universal systems of Astrology.

When I first read the book a decade ago, after finding a second-hand copy online, I was shocked that it did not have an index by default printing. I created one and realized the whole need to write this small primer.

CHAPTER NINE

A list of Herbs and their uses and classifications

Created when I found the book, Planetary Herbology by Michael Tierra, this is the index that was actually missing in it, kindly read that book for a detailed analysis.

INDEX

Warming Diaphoretics

Ephedra — lungs, bladder
Angelica — Holy Ghost Plant — "
Lovage — Love ache — "
Scallions — "
Magnolia Blossoms — lungs (causes beetle pollination in ecosystem cycle)
Hyssop — "
Sage — "
Oregano / Marjoram (Th. originally) "
Savory — "
Basil (Gk. for king) St. Joseph's Wort — "
Yerba Buena — (Esp. "Good Herb") "
Costmary — Bible leaf — Stomach & lungs
Osha — "
Hedge Nettle — "
Sassafras — "
Cinnamon

Cooling Diaphoretics

Horsemint — lungs, liver
Peppermint — "
Catnip — "
Lemon Balm "
Elder Flowers — used as a drink across Europe — "
Feverfew — "
Chrysanthemum Flowers — " (4 Chinese Gentlemen in Art. Orchid, Plum blossom & Bamboo others)

Horsetail
Duckweed

Vervain, Blue - गंधनेणु - "
Yarrow - सहस्त्रपर्णी
Pleurisy root - "
Mulberry leaves - शहतूत - "
~~Buffeum~~ Bufleurum - "
Kudzu root "
Laxatives
Rhubarb root - रेवांचीनी - Spleen, liver
Cascara Bark - "
Buck thorn Bark - झड़बेरी
Senna
Butternut/Walnut (Bark) - अखरोट
Aloe - अनार्यक
Sodium Sulphate - सेंधा
Lubricating Laxatives
Linseed - अलसी
Psyllium
Castor Oil - अरंडी का तेल
Marijuana seeds
Sesame oil - तिल का तेल
Olive oil - जैतून का तेल
Cathartic Laxatives (drastic)
Poke root - lung, kidney
Jalap - बेशरम - "
Mandrake Root
Croton Oil
Gamboge - Cambodia orange dye
Elder Bark
Scotch Broom

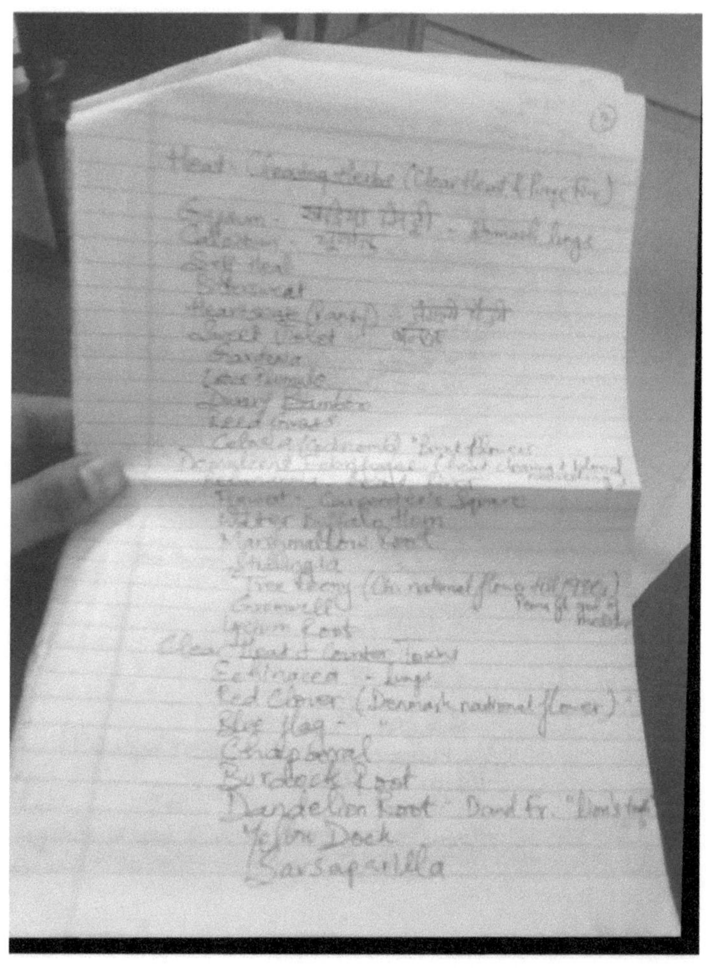
Red Clover (Denmark national flower)
Burdock Root
Yellow Dock
Sarsaparilla

Pulsatilla - Blooms near Passover
Isatis
Baptisia
Honeysuckle
Forsythia
Purslane
Bear Lichen
St John's Wort
Gotu Kola
Clear Heat + Dispell Depress
Wahoo - Burning bush liver
Willow - Symbol of death in East - "
Cinchona Bark - "
Poplar - पहाड़ी पीपल - "
Gentian - जेनशियन "
Golden Seal "
Barberry "
Oregon Grape - "
Boldo - Lt America growth only - "
Fringetree - "
Bitterroot -
Culver's Root
Fumitory
Centaury
Cascara Amarga
Greater Celandine
Clear Summer Heat (Weather Induced)
Hibiscus - गुड़हल
Borage - पत्थरचूर
Hound's tongue - Sticks to wool of sheep, causes photosensitivity on ingestion by them

Mung Bean
Southernwood / Wormwood, Common
Watermelon
Cucumber
Lotus Leaf
Impatiens (Jewelweed) · Touch me not, Balsam
Diuretics (Regulation of Water Metabolism)

Poria - Bladder
Dandelion leaf
Parsley [illegible] अजमोद
Coriander धनिया
Buchu
Plantain - [illegible]
Gravel Root
Cleavers
Hydrangea
Pellitory of the wall
Water Plantain - [illegible]
Couchgrass
Wild Carrot Queen Anne's Lace (N. Amr)
Knotweed -
Watermelon Seed
Uva ursi - Bear Berry
Pipsissewa · Prince's pine
Watercress - [illegible]
Azuki Bean (Aduki Bean) [illegible]
Corn Silk - Maize flower
Antirheumatic (Dispelling wind & Dampness)
Guiacam - National tree of Bahamas · [illegible]
Polypody fern

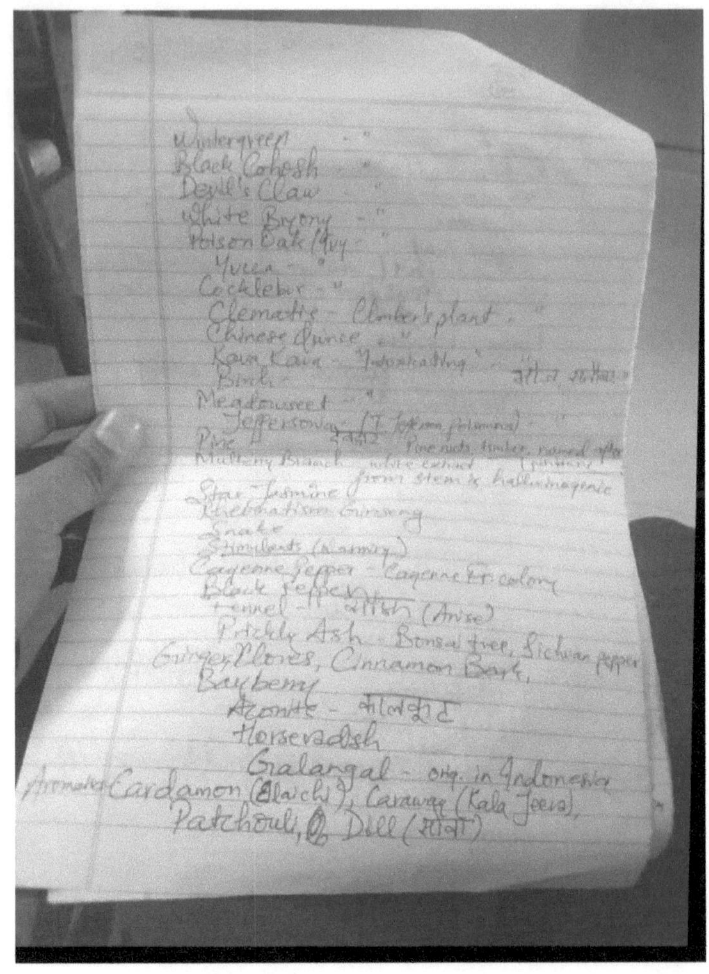
Wintergreen - "
Black Cohosh - "
Devil's Claw - "
White Bryony - "
Poison Oak (Ivy - "
Yucca - "
Cocklebur - "
Clematis - Climber's plant - "
Chinese Quince - "
Birch -
Meadowsweet - "
Pine
Star Jasmine
Snake
Cayenne Pepper - Cayenne Fr. colony
Black Pepper
Fennel - सौंफ (Anise)
Prickly Ash - Bonsai tree, Sichuan pepper
Ginger, Cloves, Cinnamon Bark,
Bayberry
Aconite - कालकूट
Horseradish
Galangal - orig. in Indonesia
Cardamon (Elaichi), Caraway (Kala Jeera),
Patchouli, Dill (सोवा)

Carminatives (Regulators of Chi)

3 Citrus - Orange peel digestion, Green Orange Peel - bile to liver
(Chinese) Bitter orange for abdominal indigestion

Cyperus (Sedge root)
Sandalwood - चंदन
Chinese Chive - Manipuri term is Maroinakup
Persimmon Calyx
Cumin (जीरा)
Digestants
Hawthorn berry
Barley
Hemostatics (regulating blood)
Raspberry leaves
Agrimony
Mugwort
Thuja - देवदार leaves
Cattail pollen
thistles
Shepherd's Purse
Burnet Root
Lotus nodes
Trillium (Ontario National flower)
Ginseng
Blood Vitalizers - Emmenagogues
Corydalis (Turkey corn)
Turmeric
Motherwort
Bugleweed
Peach : आडू

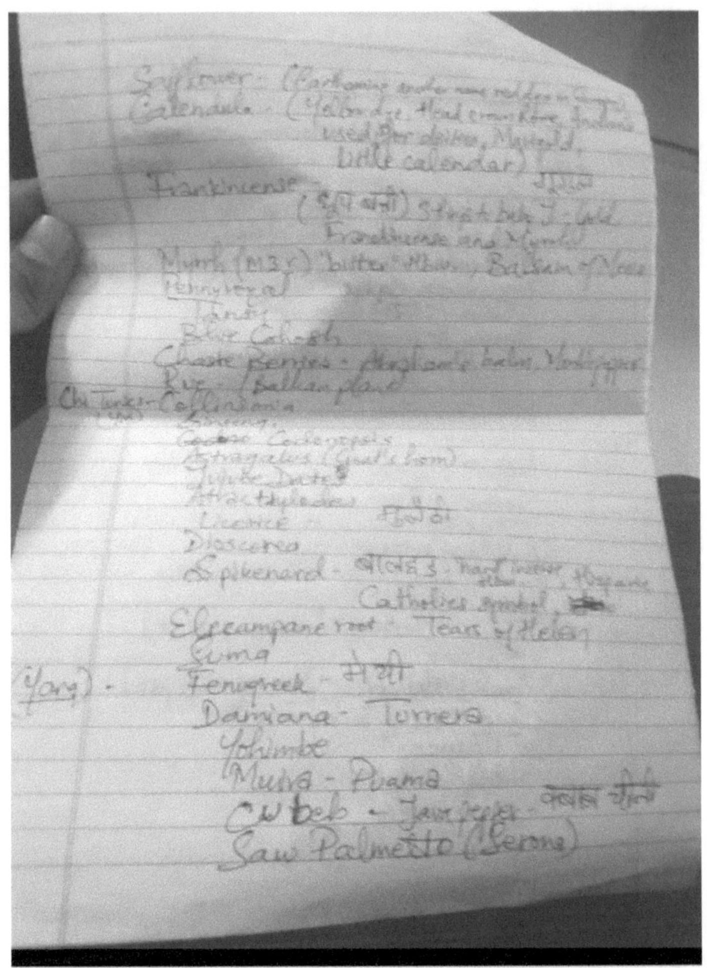

Calendula
little calendar)
Frankincense
Frankincense and Myrrh
Myrrh
Blue Cohosh
Chaste Berries
Astragalus
Jujube Dates
Atractylodes
Licorice
Dioscorea
Spikenard
Catholics symbol
Elecampane root - Tears of Helen
Suma
Fenugreek - मेथी
Damiana - Turnera
Yohimbe
Muira - Puama
Cubeb - Java pepper
Saw Palmetto (Serenoa)

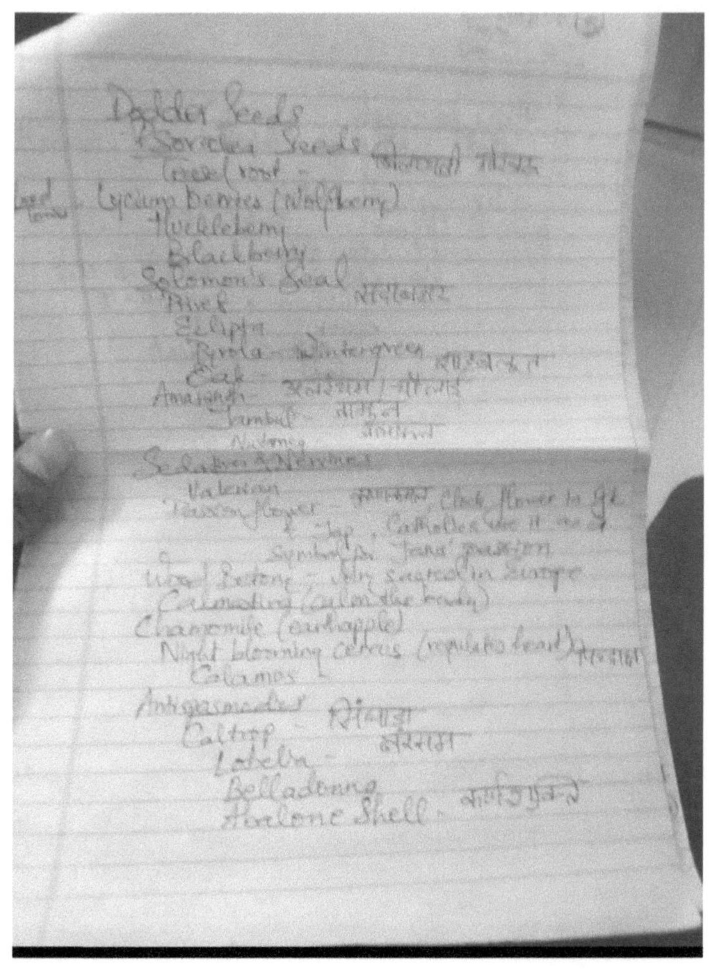
Dodder Seeds
Lycium berries (Wolfberry)
Huckleberry
Blackberry
Solomon's Seal
Eclipta
Pyrola - Wintergreen
Valerian
Passion flower
Chamomile (earthapple)
Night blooming cereus (regulates heart)
Calamus
Caltrop - सिंघाड़ा
Lobelia
Belladonna
Abalone Shell

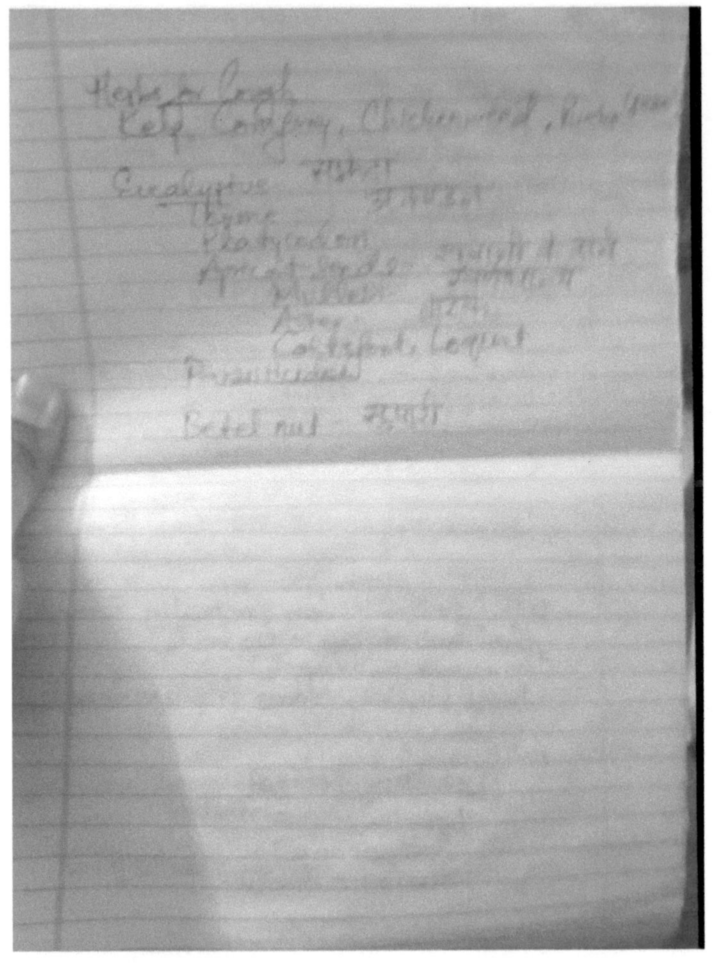

CHAPTER TEN

The demand for AYUSH in times of troubling events in Allopathy

I seek to make only two points. Even though our healthcare infrastructure in India is bad, our doctors remain one of the best in Allopathy. There are two things that are paramount requiring revision in our legal and on-ground structures.

The first is the problem outlined in the book Heart Mafia by Biswaroop Chowdhury. Not only is a heart problem getting rampantly created along with Diabetes due to rash and loud driving of upper than 100cc bikes and vehicles without silencers, but that is also only alluded to by the author. All countries to our West starting from Pakistan to Iran do not allow this to happen. Then, the belief that Heart problems occur due to a certain lifestyle that is associated with the privileged becomes a political license to war. A disease is a disease and it must be cured using minimum resources for all. A law on loud vehicles must be enforced, as with the passage of time, such ailments are natural to grow, as can be viewed in a Medical statistics for Hypertension and Diabetes across the recent decades.

The second is the problem outlined in Dinesh Thakur's book The Truth Pill and although he has been fighting the legal and executive system for a long, the problem of counterfeit and poisonous drugs continues. Recently an African country sent back cough syrups that killed several dozen kids in their country. We must heed his word, as the government of India is constantly prey to severe criticism here.

The third, a positive message in a gloomy time, is that at the time of genetic engineering and completed test tube babies, the direction is forward and not towards anti-vaccines and anti-allopathy because as the world progresses, pollutes and develops, the direction is towards exo-planet inhabitation and not just sustainable and eco-friendly production.

9 798888 695548

Printed by Libri Plureos GmbH in Hamburg, Germany